Manuel Díaz Curiel
Rosa Arboiro Pinel

Primary hyperparathyroidism

Manuel Díaz Curiel
Rosa Arboiro Pinel

Primary hyperparathyroidism

ScienciaScripts

Imprint

Any brand names and product names mentioned in this book are subject to trademark, brand or patent protection and are trademarks or registered trademarks of their respective holders. The use of brand names, product names, common names, trade names, product descriptions etc. even without a particular marking in this work is in no way to be construed to mean that such names may be regarded as unrestricted in respect of trademark and brand protection legislation and could thus be used by anyone.

Cover image: www.ingimage.com

This book is a translation from the original published under ISBN 978-613-9-43719-1.

Publisher:
Sciencia Scripts
is a trademark of
Dodo Books Indian Ocean Ltd. and OmniScriptum S.R.L publishing group

120 High Road, East Finchley, London, N2 9ED, United Kingdom
Str. Armeneasca 28/1, office 1, Chisinau MD-2012, Republic of Moldova, Europe
Printed at: see last page
ISBN: 978-620-7-15164-6

TABLE OF CONTENTS

Chapter 1   **6**

Chapter 2   **20**

Chapter 3   **29**

PRIMARY HYPERPARATHYROIDISM

Dr Manuel Diaz Curiel, Dr Rosa Arboiro Pinel
Department of Internal Medicine/ Metabolic Bone Diseases
Fundacion Jimenez Diaz Madrid

DEFINITION AND HISTORY

Primary hyperparathyroidism (PHP) is the most common endocrine disease after diabetes mellitus (1 in 1500 hospital admissions) in adulthood as its age of presentation coincides with the second half of life(38). It is a clinical situation in which there is excessive secretion of PTH by the parathyroid glands, leading to chronic hypercalcaemia and alterations in the hormone's main target organs (kidney and bone)(5,6). It is the most frequent cause of hypercalcaemia in non-hospitalised patients(5,27).

The first description of PPH was made in 1705, in an inhabitant of the city of Sedan, by the Frenchman Courtial.(54) However, it was not until the end of the 19th century that the typical picture began to be defined with the description of the association of osteopathy with nephrocalcinosis by Davies-Colley in 1884, and the characteristic cystic fibrous osteitis by Von Recklinghausen in 1891. The first tumour of the parathyroid glands was found in 1904 by Azkanazy, who removed them at autopsy from a deceased patient with Recklinhausen's bone disease. In 1925 Mandi removed the first parathyroid tumour from a patient y Charles Martell was the first patient studied for PPH, with a diffuse bone process and alterations in calcium metabolism, and was operated on in May 1926 at the Massachusetts Hospital, a year after Mandi's first intervention. The tumour, however, was not found until the patient's seventh operation six years later. This was the first stage of PPH, which we can call the osseous stage, to which the renal stage was then added, which was due to Albright(1). This same author, in 1941, made the first description of an ectopic PTH-secreting tumour. In the same year, he was the first to draw attention to the prevalence of osteoporosis of the spine in postmenopausal women.

In 1954 Seidinger performed the first arteriographic localisation of a parathyroid adenoma. In 1963, Berson, Yalow and Auerbach performed the first radioimmunoassay (RIA) for human bovine PTH, which was used clinically from 1966. In the following years, progress has been made in the knowledge and identification by RIA of the PTH molecule and its different fragments, in the characterisation of the disease, its medical treatment, techniques for non-invasive localisation of the pathological gland and in the genetic abnormalities underlying different forms of PPH(5,54).

PREVALENCE AND INCIDENCE

The prevalence of the disease is estimated to be up to 0.2% in patients over 60 years of age, with an estimated prevalence in asymptomatic, undiscovered subjects of 0.1% or higher. The generalisation of automated serum calcium determinations has increased the recognition of PPH, especially in elderly patients(20).

The age-adjusted annual incidence of PPH in the general population is estimated to be around 25 cases per 100,000 population. The incidence in women over 60 years of age is 188 cases per 100,000 and 92 cases per 100,000 in men, while the incidence in men and women under 39 years of age is less than 10 cases per 100,000.

with exceptional cases in children. In our experience, 63% of patients were over 70 years of age, and 90% were over 50 years of age. The female/male ratio was 7:1 in the age group over 70 years(42).

AETIOPATHOGENESIS/ MOLECULAR BASIS OF HPP

The cause of most parathyroid tumours is not known although their association with previous ionising neck irradiation has been described while their higher incidence in postmenopausal women would suggest a tumourogenesis o promotion of the clinical expression of previous silent PPH, in relation to oestrogen deficiency(5,25).

In recent decades there has been great interest in the hereditary aspects of PPH **(TABLE I),** sometimes associated with other endocrine diseases, notably multiple endocrine neoplasia (MEN) type I and type **11(3).**

The molecular mechanisms involved in the development of parathyroid tumours confirm the monoclonality of adenomas although it has also been described in cases of primary or secondary hyperplasia(56).

Recognition of the monoclonality of parathyroid adenomas led to the suspicion that this type of tumour, despite its mostly benign nature, followed the general principles of tumour genesis described for most tumours (somatic involvement, need for multiple mutations, monoclonality, genes restricted to a few tumour types y genes involved in multiple types).

In recent years, several molecular genetic mechanisms involved in the genesis of parathyroid neoplasms have been described. This has made it possible to confirm the monoclonal origin of parathyroid neoplasms, to better understand the pathogenic mechanisms involved in tumour genesis, as well as the implications for diagnosis, prognosis and treatment that the development of simpler and faster techniques for the detection of these genetic alterations may have in the future, especially in cases of MEN and parathyroid carcinoma.

Loss of function of at least one tumour suppressor gene usually contributes to 25% of non-familial parathyroid adenomas. Rearrangement y overexpression of the proto-oncogene PRAD1 (cyclin 1), inactivation of a tumour suppressor gene on chromosome 11; reported in most cases of MEN type I (llql3 region) while MEN type II is found on the pericentromeric region of chromosome 10 (10qll.2 region). Both can be the cause of sporadic parathyroid adenoma presentation. The tumour suppressor gene involved in retinoblastoma, described on chromosome 13, may be a factor in the pathogenesis of parathyroid carcinoma(35).

The mutation in the calcium-sensitive receptor gene (a member of the G-protein-binding receptor superfamily), now responsible for familial hypocalciuric hypercalcaemia, familial benign hypercalcaemia and severe neonatal PPH, is located on the long arm of chromosome 3 (3q2).

Chapter 1

<u>**PATHOLOGICAL ANATOMY**</u>

The clinical pathological classification y the aetiology of PPH is controversial y most of the glands analysed in PPH show nodular or diffuse hyperplasia when carefully analysed by histological techniques(lO).

In fact, it is impossible to distinguish adenoma from hyperplasia by histological examination of a single gland and it is difficult to decide by objective criteria whether these abnormalities occur in one or all four glands. In any case, if only one gland is affected, its resection is followed by cure of the disease, while recurrence is equally rare.

PARATHYROID ADENOMA (in 80% of PPH cases):

<u>- Single adenoma</u>. It is a benign, well encapsulated tumour of variable weight (between 0.2-15 g), size and shape (usually ovoid), dark orange in colour and soft in consistency. The normal gland contains abundant parenchymal fat, which is usually found in only 50-60% of cases.

Adenomas are usually composed of principal cells, with a slightly eosinophilic cytoplasm and a round, central nucleus and occasionally hyperchromatic and even mitotically active, as in other benign endocrine neoplasms. In other cases there are oxyphilic cells, clear cells or a mixture of these.

Immunochemical studies positive for chromogranin, parathormone antibodies, and negative for thyroglobulin, calcitonin or thyroid follicular epithelium are useful for differential diagnosis with other tumours of thyroid origin.

<u>- Multiple parathyroid adenomas</u>. Double adenomas are rare y corresponding to pseudoadenomatous o asymmetric hyperplasia.

<u>**HYPERPLASIA PARATIRQIDEA** (in 13%):</u>

The most common is primary principal cell hyperplasia with an increase in the overall mass of the four glands in the absence of an external stimulus of parathormone hypersecretion. It is therefore essential to study at least two glands to confirm the diagnosis. It has also been called nodular hyperplasia or multiple adenomatosis.

Three histological patterns have been described: the classic, with homogeneous involvement of all four glands, the pseudoadenomatous pattern with variations in the size of the glands; and the "occult" form, in which the glands are apparently normal with only histological evidence of hyperplasia.

The predominant cellularity is principal cells although oncocytic cells are occasionally seen, y fatty stromal decrease y nodular presentation. Occasionally nuclear pleomorphic mitosis is seen, although this is more a finding in adenomas.

Less common is tiara cell hyperplasia, for some with a personality of its own, where all four glands are affected with cells whose cytoplasm has a clear appearance filled with small vacuoles, probably derived from Golgi vesicles.

<u>**PARATHYROID CARCINOMA:**</u>

Parathyroid carcinoma, described in 2 % of PPH cases, is characterised by a large size (mean weight 12 grams) with a trabecular alignment of tumour cells divided by fibrous bands. There is usually capsular and vascular invasion and mitotic figures are easily found.

Pathological diagnosis poses serious problems, as the usual criteria for malignancy, as in other endocrine tumours, do not have the same value in carcinoma.

Histopathological criteria for diagnosis have been established with thick fibrous bands, mitotic activity, capsular and vascular invasion. The finding of aneuploid cells by flow cytometry to measure DNA content is often helpful in this diagnosis. Especially if an S-phase fraction greater than 4 per cent and a DNA index greater than 1.2 are found (35).

Depending on the parathyroid embryology, there are usually ectopic parathyroid glands, so adenomas located in the upper mediastinum, within the thymus, behind the oesophagus or intra-thyroid have been described; they are found in no more than 10% of cases.

There is a frequent association of PPH with other thyroid and extra-thyroid neoplasms, which appears to be greater than chance(38).

Marked differences in clinical appearance have been described depending on the histopathology of the parathyroid gland. Patients with large adenomas generally have more pronounced hypercalcaemia and more severe bone disease, whereas hyperplasia is associated with younger male patients with renal lithiasis and less hypercalcaemia. It has also been observed that the neuromuscular and psychiatric forms are more frequent in older women with high calcaemia values, often coinciding with adenomas.

PHYSIOPATOLOGIA.

In all forms of PPH there are three pathophysiological mechanisms that contribute to varying degrees to PTH hypersecretion: there is a change in the calcium sensor tipping point, a higher proportion of active cells reflects the increased secretory activity, and thirdly, there is an increase in the total number of parenchymal cells. However, there is no direct correlation between gland weight, PTH values or hypercalcaemia values, explaining the variability of biochemical and clinical parameters among patients with PPH (6).

The secretion of other substances by parathyroid tumours has also been confirmed сото chromogranin A o PSP-1(49), protein II o parathyroid hypertensive factor(44).

NATURAL HISTORY AND CLINICAL PICTURE

The following clinical forms are usually distinguished:

- PPH accompanied by renal lithiasis: This is the most frequent form in our environment (38%). Its incidence has decreased in relation to the change in the approach to its therapeutic solution following the appearance of external lithotripsy.

- Hypercalcaemic PPH (22%): Includes patients with any symptoms associated with hypercalcaemia.

- PPH associated with bone pathology (10%): This corresponds to the initially described form сото fibrosing osteitis, although the progressive association with osteoporosis would make it necessary to include this disease among the bone forms.

- Asymptomatic PPH (15%): This is the hypercalcaemic form that presents without clinical manifestations and is mainly detected in people over 60 years of age.

- PPH normocalcaemic (8%): Intermittent hypercalcaemia or sustained normocalcaemia y whose only manifestation is usually renal lithiasis.

- Familial PPH (7%): When there is a family history of the same disease, including MEN.

The clinical spectrum of PPH has changed considerably in recent years(34,55). It has shifted from presenting manifestations typical of severe bone and kidney disease to apparently asymptomatic disease with vague symptoms.

The reasons for this change include demographic changes (PPH is mainly a disease of middle-aged or elderly adults), diffusion of medical knowledge leading to a higher index of suspicion and technological improvement of the clinical laboratory(24).

One of the most important aspects has been the changes in the clinical presentation of this disease, as shown in **TABLE II, which** confirms a progressive decrease in the bone and hypercalcaemic forms. More accurate biochemical data have recently led to the disappearance of the well-known form como "normocalcaemic" PPH. The diagnosis of asymptomatic PPH has gradually increased and the other clinical forms of presentation have remained stable over time(42).

Since PPH was first described, attention has been drawn to the presentation of two main clinical forms: one with renal involvement and the other with mainly bone involvement. There are several pathogenic theories to explain this dual presentation of PPH: the existence of a "double hormone", the size of the parathyroid tumour and the serum values of $1,25(OH)_2 D_3$, since in cases where these are elevated, PPH manifests with hypercalciuria, which would favour the development of renal lithiasis(6).

a)   . - BONE DISEASE

Bone involvement in PPH has been recognised since the disease was first described as one of its main clinical manifestations. Although many patients with PPH have histological changes in bone, these are clinically apparent in only a relatively small number of patients. Skeletal changes are varied. They are rarely severe, with bone pain, deformity, bone cysts and susceptibility to fractures. This is the classic PPH bone disease, fibrous cystic osteitis (FCO), first described a hundred years ago (1). Nowadays it is a rare form of presentation of PPH. At the time of diagnosis, severe bone disease with symptoms is present in less than 15% of patients and radiological CFO is currently present in less than 5%. The reason why CBO is an unusual coтo form of disease presentation is because PPH is diagnosed, by routine serum calcium determinations, at an earlier stage of the disease. However, many patients with PPH often have diffuse vertebral osteopenia at presentation, and this is a much more frequent manifestation than CBO. The bone involvement that we see most often in clinical practice today is diffuse osteoporosis (18).

Clinically and radiologically, three forms of bone involvement are seen in PPH: osteitis fibrosa, osteoporosis and osteosclerosis(6).

- <u>Osteitis fibrosquamous</u> is characterised by the following lesions:

- Subperiosteal bone resorption: usually seen at the level of the phalanges, acromioclavicular joints, pubic symphysis and sacroiliac joints. Subperiosteal resorption is most frequently and best seen at the level of the lateral sides of the middle and distal phalanges. The earliest lesions are seen near the base of the phalanx y are localised. Similar lesions often appear on the skull, which acquires a "salt and pepper" appearance. Another characteristic localisation of radiographic changes is at the level of the distal third of the clavicle.

- Loss of dental hard laminae: Characteristic but not specific.

- Cystic lesions: Two types of cystic lesions are seen in patients with PPH, true bone cysts and brown tumours. On radiographic study they have a similar appearance, and are often difficult to distinguish. Bone cysts are occupied by fibrous tissue and have a subperiosteal location. They do not resolve after surgical treatment of PPH. In contrast, brown tumours are occupied by osteoclasts and osteoblasts, forming poorly mineralised bone. They are known as osteoclastomas. These lesions resolve when PPH is successfully treated surgically **(15).**

- Osteoporosis. In recent literature, much attention has been devoted to the determination of bone mass in patients with PPH, with the aim of clarifying which type of bone or skeletal region is most affected in this disease, what is the speed and significance of this bone loss, and whether this is in any way relevant to a decision on surgical treatment.

Decreased bone mineral density (BMD) is a known complication of PPH and is usually asymptomatic for a long period of time until fracture occurs, so bone mass measurement is indicated in the initial evaluation of the patient with PPH, even if asymptomatic, since PPH patients lose bone at different rates in different parts of the skeleton, so bone mass measurement in one bone does not predict bone loss at another level (12).

Since the introduction of densitometry techniques, several studies have demonstrated the existence of a loss of BMD in patients with PPH when compared with a similar age group and it is known that this bone loss is not homogeneous throughout the skeleton. With a prevalence in patients under 60 years of age of 5.9% and 8.4% in those over 60 years of age **(TABLE III).**

In relation to the type of bone affected in patients with PPH, greater bone loss has been observed in cortical bone, which is predominantly in the peripheral skeleton, as this bone appears to be more sensitive to the effect of PTH. Bone loss is not always homogeneous, as it can occur in specific locations such as the skull, phalanges and clavicles. While the involvement of trabecular bone, predominantly in the spine, is less severe and of later onset, which would explain a higher incidence of vertebral crushing in PPH **(4).**

- Osteosclerosis: Osteosclerosis, which is usually diffuse or localised, is much more frequent (5-20%) in hyperparathyroidism secondary to chronic renal failure. In cases of PPH in children, osteosclerosis of the metaphyseal regions of rapidly growing bones is typical. Osteosclerosis usually occurs as a result of the anabolic effects of PTH on the skeleton **(18).**

b)   . - RENAL INVOLVEMENT:

Renal involvement is, after asymptomatic cases, the most common form of PPH. It includes anatomical and functional changes, including nephrolithiasis, nephrocalcinosis, decreased glomerular filtration rate and various tubular abnormalities resulting from hypercalcaemia and elevated PTH.

- <u>Renal lithiasis</u> is the predominant clinical syndrome, with PPH being the second leading cause of calcium stones. Due to the decreasing prevalence of stone disease and the fact that most kidney stones disappear quickly and are too small to cause urinary tract obstruction, the number of patients with PPH and kidney stones requiring surgical treatment has decreased.

The incidence of renal lithiasis in PPH ranges from 18% to 46.7%. The usual composition of calculi is calcium phosphate or a mixture of phosphate and calcium oxalate, with hypercalciuria and alkalinuria being important in their pathogenesis. All patients with confirmed PPH should be checked for the possible presence of urolithiasis. In 5-10% of patients with recurrent calcific lithiasis, PPH is usually found. In patients treated with lithotripsy, a prevalence of PPH of 1.65% to 3.02% is observed. Generally, patients with renal lithiasis do not have bone involvement.

Differences have been observed in the prevalence of renal lithiasis in PPH, according to age and sex. Thus, a higher prevalence of renal lithiasis is found in men (58%) than in women (28%), and in young people under 50 years of age with slight hypercalcaemia (87%), than in older people with higher calcium values (30%). A higher prevalence has also been observed in patients with primary cell hyperplasia than in those with adenoma **(51)**.

Hypocitraturia is a potential cause of calcium lithiasis, because citrate reduces the concentration of calcium ion in renal tubular fluid and thus reduces the risk of calcium precipitation and the formation of kidney stones. Patients with PPH associated with renal lithiasis, but without bone involvement, have marked hypocitraturia (urinary citrate <320 mg/day o urinary citrate/creatinine ratio<0.200), due to increased tubular citrate reabsorption. However, patients with renal lithiasis o bone involvement have hypercalciuria o normocitraturia o hypercitraturia, as do patients with exclusively bone involvement. These data postulate the involvement of citrate in the presentation of renal lithiasis in PPH (2).

- <u>Nephrocalcinosis</u> is more frequent, due to the fact that the diagnosis of PPH is nowadays made at earlier stages of the disease. Thus, it is generally observed that its incidence has decreased from 22% (between 1930-60) to 3% (between 1972-81). It usually occurs in patients with severe, long-standing disease, with significant impairment of glomerular filtration and tubular function. It is due to precipitation of calcium and phosphate in the renal tubular epithelium and renal interstitial tissue. It is sometimes difficult to determine whether renal failure is a consequence o cause of nephrocalcinosis. Increased serum phosphorus, which occurs coto consequence of impaired glomerular filtration, is necessary for the precipitation of calcium phosphate salts in the renal parenchyma, which often further impairs renal function. Nephrocalcinosis is most frequently seen in patients with bone involvement and parathyroid carcinoma.

- Of the functional alterations, the most common is <u>renal tubular acidosis</u>. PTH acts at the proximal tubule level by inhibiting bicarbonate reabsorption, causing increased bicarbonate elimination and hyperchloremic acidosis. In addition to renal tubular acidosis there is often also phosphaturia, aminoaciduria y glucosuria, all of which are consequences of a direct effect of PTH on the proximal tubule. Decreased phosphate reabsorption is the predominant effect of PTH at the proximal tubular level. In addition to these effects there is a decrease in the ability to concentrate urine, probably due to tubular resistance to ADH. The pathogenesis of changes in renal tubular function is complex. They are usually due to a direct effect of PTH or hypercalcaemia, or a combination of both.

- The most important functional disorder is <u>renal insufficiency</u> with retention of nitrogenous products, a consequence of volume depletion which, due to altered urine concentration, causes hypercalcaemia. There are also cases of impaired filtration secondary to the structural abnormalities described above, as these lead to interstitial nephritis.

c)   . - OTHER MANIFESTATIONS:

<u>-Neuromuscular</u> complications The neuromuscular syndrome associated with PPH consists of proximal muscle weakness, easy fatigue and atrophy due to denervation of type II muscle fibres. Patients show a loss of limb root strength with characteristic difficulty in standing, walking and raising the arms. A higher prevalence has been observed in women (25%) than in men (10%).

Electromyographic alterations include shortening of the duration of potentials with decreased amplitude, presence of peripheral potentials and preserved conduction velocity. Smooth muscle involvement often leads to hypomotility of the colon and consequent strenulation.

<u>-Psychiatric</u> complications This presentation is described with increasing frequency (between 39 y 45%), with an important difference to the older series described(22).

There are usually symptoms of fatigue, weakness, irritability, sleep disturbances, anxiety, lack of concentration and memory that are prevalent in the general population, but non-specific and difficult to quantify. Psychiatric manifestations including depression, personality changes or psychosis have also been described. The prevalence of these symptoms is 23%, predominantly in older patients, with depression and anxiety being the most frequent disorders (7).

In patients with severe hypercalcaemia who usually present clinically with lethargy, stupor and eventually coma (52).

- Gastrointestinal manifestations of PPH are usually subtle, such as vague abdominal discomfort, o secondary to hypercalcaemia, como anorexia, nausea, diffuse abdominal pain, weight loss o and constipation; o or they are often manifested by disturbances of the stomach o and pancreas(5,25).

Peptic ulcus is particularly common in PPH, although it is not clear whether there is a causal relationship between the two entities or whether it is a fortuitous association of two relatively common diseases in the general population. The incidence of peptic ulcus varies from 4.8% to 16%, with no significant differences according to the age of the patients.

The interrelationship between calcaemia and serum gastrin concentrations is important. Hypercalcaemia induces an increase in gastrin and basal C1H hypersecretion. Thus, the incidence of duodenal ulcer in PPH may be mediated by the effect of PTH and calcium on gastrin. Chronic hypercalcaemia, whether of parathyroid origin or not, usually increases gastrin values (up to 22% of patients), although very high values are indicative of Zollinger Ellison syndrome, associated with MEN type I **(49).**

Abdominal pain is usually due to hypertonia of the gastrointestinal tract due to decreased muscle excitability due to hypercalcaemia or pancreatitis. The association between acute pancreatitis and PPH is clear but rare (2-7%). This association is 6-10 times higher in acute PPH than in chronic PPH. In some patients, acute pancreatitis is often the presenting form of PPH.

Eighty per cent of patients with PPH and associated pancreatitis have serum calcium values above 12 mg/dl and in 30% of cases it is associated with renal lithiasis. In 30% of cases, pancreatitis is acute, while in 34% it is chronic. In the remaining third, episodes of pancreatitis are recurrent. Acute necrotic-hemorrhagic pancreatitis occurs predominantly in the course of hypercalcaemic crises with a mortality rate of 40%.

- Joint complications Several joint complications have been described in PPH: chondrocalcinosis, gout, degenerative osteoarthritis, ankylosing spondylitis and tendon avulsion.

Chondrocalcinosis: Also known as pseudogout, it is a clinical entity characterised by the presence of arthritis and pain in one or more joints associated with the presence of calcium pyrophosphate dihydrate crystals in the synovial fluid. Their radiological presence is estimated at 18% y 40%, with a predominance in older patients. In addition to the clinical presentation of arthritis, radiological findings are suggestive of the diagnosis, such as the aspiration of joint fluid and the demonstration of weakly positive birefringence on microscopic examination. The most commonly affected joints are knees and elbows. 10-20% of patients usually have joint calcification or fibrocartilage calcification, especially at the meniscus and the triangular cartilage of the wrist. The differential diagnosis with calcifications of degenerative arthropathies is made by the absence of degenerative changes in the neighbouring bone.

Gout: Hyperuricaemia is common in patients with PPH, due to decreased renal clearance of urate. Acute episodes of gout are not uncommon in patients with PPH, with a frequency of 57.6%. The most commonly affected joints are those of the lower extremities, with characteristic localisation in the first metatarsophalangeal joint. Gout and chondrocalcinosis often occur together in the same patient, and 20% of patients with pseudogout also have hyperuricaemia. Gout and chondrocalcinosis differ in the type of joint affected, the severity of pain in gout, the presence of mono-sodium urate crystals in the joint fluid, which show a strong birefringence on microscopic examination, and the characteristic response of gouty arthritis to colchicine.

- <u>Metastatic calcifications In</u> addition to nephrocalcinosis and chondrocalcinosis, calcifications may occur in other tissues such as the lungs, arteries, heart, pituitary gland, liver and skeletal muscle. In the cornea there is precipitation of calcium and phosphate crystals, leading to band keratopathy, which is the most typical ocular manifestation of PPH.

Calcifications also often occur at the skin level, due to precipitation of calcium and phosphate in the subcutaneous tissue and epidermis, causing pruritus and skin necrosis; this is more common in secondary hyperparathyroidism(18).

- <u>Cardiovascular involvement In terms</u> of cardiac involvement in PPH, a high incidence (68%) of left ventricular hypertrophy, calcification of the aortic and/or mitral valves (63-49%) and calcification of the myocardium have been observed. One year after parathyroid dectomy and restoration of normocalcaemia, regression of cardiac hypertrophy is observed while calcifications persist, with no evidence of progression **(53).**

Arterial hypertension complicates the prognosis of PPH through several mechanisms, since clinical factors are involved, such as the age of presentation and female preference, renal failure, hypercalcaemic nephropathy or nephrocalcinosis, as well as other pathogenic disorders, such as the renin-angiotensin system, serum PTH values and mobilisation of sodium deposited in the bone. However, the most important factor is hypercalcaemia itself, which increases cardiac contractility and secondarily vasomotor tone with a consequent increase in blood pressure. PPH is often part of an MEN which includes other diseases with hypertension, such as Cushing's syndrome, pheochromocytoma or, more rarely, hyperaldosteronism.

Several studies have found hypertension to be more frequent in asymptomatic PPH than in controls (26.3% vs. 15.5%) **(39)**. At the same time, a normalisation of blood pressure after parathyroidectomy has been reported, so that hypertension has been advocated as an indication for surgery, even in subjects with asymptomatic PPH. The role played by the parathyroid hypertensive factor(44) is still under study.

- Endocrine manifestations Hypercalcaemia induces alterations in the activity of other hormone receptors, a reversible phenomenon after removal of the responsible tumour. Thus, hypergastrinaemia or hydrocarbon intolerance have been described, which are reversible after removal of the tumour responsible. In other cases, PPH is part of the endocrine constellation of MEN (27).

Chapter 2

SIGNS AND SYMPTOMS

The clinical features of PPH are derived from hypercalcaemia. In other cases, hypercalcaemia is asymptomatic o with unremarkable symptoms, so that surgical intervention cannot be expected to solve all the problems arising from the patient's symptoms **(33).**

In general, symptoms usually affect the gastrointestinal tract (anorexia, nausea, vomiting, constipation, indefinite abdominal pain; all accompanied by weight loss); the renal system with polyuria, polydipsia, nocturia, dehydration, nephrolithiasis, nephrocalcinosis, neuromuscular and skeletal symptoms with back and limb pain, muscle weakness, lethargy, vasomotor instability, and the central nervous system is often affected, ranging from laxity to confusion, instability, memory loss, decreased visual acuity, somnolence, stupor and coma(38).

<u>Familial PPH</u> Although PPH most often occurs sporadically, several types of familial PPH are currently described **(TABLE I).** These include familial PPH associated with MEN, type I y II, familial isolated PPH and familial hypocalciuric hypercalcaemia which is an autosomal dominant disease characterised by calcium receptor insensitivity with altered PTH secretion turning point and decreased urinary calcium excretion **(30).**

PHYSICAL EXAMINATION

Physical examination does not provide any interesting data in these patients, except for the finding of corneal calcifications or sclerotic calcifications and arterial hypertension, a common finding at this age of disease presentation, especially in women. Palpation of the responsive tumour in the neck is a frequent finding, less than 1%, given the small size of the tumour. In cases of neuromuscular involvement, myopathic symptomatology or data consistent with cerebral complications of acute hypercalcaemia may be observed (36). Bone fractures with visible deformities or loss of height in relation to vertebral fractures are associated with osteoporosis. In the case of subperiosteal resorption of the phalanges, the fingers are reminiscent of a "drumstick".

GENERAL BIOCHEMISTRY (TABLE IV)

PPH is the most frequent cause of hypercalcaemia in the outpatient setting (more than 85%).

In PPH, hypophosphataemia is related to parathyroid hyperfunction, as renal tubular phosphorus handling is regulated by PTH, which leads to a reduction in renal tubular reabsorption (RTP).

RTP is found to be decreased in PPH although its value is low in the presence of renal failure. Other more subtle determinations, como the phosphate/GFR TM, do not improve the diagnosis.

The plasma chloride/phosphorus ratio could facilitate the differential diagnosis of hypercalcaemia, being elevated in PPH and normal in other non-parathyroid causes of hypercalcaemia (11).

OTHER BIOCHEMICAL DATA

 - Hormonal

<u>Nephrogenic tic-AMP.</u> The effect of PTH is mediated by cAMP through a mechanism involving the receptor y a G-protein. PTH interacts with its receptors on the contraluminal membrane by acting on membrane adenylyl cyclase. cAMP binds to the regulatory subunit of the luminal membrane-dependent cAMP-dependent protein kinase by scavenging the catalytic subunit of the enzyme.

Luminal membrane proteins are phosphorylated resulting in inhibition of phosphorus and sodium cotransport.

The cAMP, acting as a second messenger, can serve as a diagnostic for PPH. Of all circulating cAMP, which is therefore influenced by other hormones, particularly catecholamines, the fraction we are interested in is that generated in the kidney itself, which is exclusively stimulated by PTH. Therefore, from the total circulating cAMP, we assess the nephrogenic cAMP, which provides a high specificity for the diagnosis of PPH, since above 60% the diagnosis of PPH can be affirmed.

<u>Vitamin D and its metabolites.</u> Vitamin D and its metabolites are of interest for the differential diagnosis of hypercalcaemia. Since vitamin D is stimulated by PTH, in cases of PPH, its mean values have been reported to be higher than normal.

In the past, two types of PPH were considered to exist, one in relation to $1,25(OH)_2 D_3$ and the other in relation to normal $1,25(OH)_2 D_3$, thus defining the renal forms from the bone forms. Today, this distinction is academic and has no other aim than the possibility of medical treatment of PPH with vitamin D in cases where the vitamin D level is low (13).

b)   Non-hormonal

<u>Calciuria:</u> PTH causes an increase in tubular reabsorption of calcium, so calcium should decrease in the urine in PPH. But in hypercalcaemia, the increased calcium filtered through the glomerulus leads to hypercalciuria. Therefore the result of both factors

contradictory conditions the appearance of calcium in the urine which is only elevated in 56% of men and 59% of women with PPH.

If stricter indices of renal tubular calcium handling are used, coтo is the rate of calcium excretion is elevated in 71.8% of males y in 74.6% of females. This conditions the relative diagnosis of hypercalciuria and incidence of lithiasis in PPH **(6).**

Two types have been reported in the clinical presentation of PPH, one with renal lithiasis and the other with preferential bone manifestation, the urinary calcium being elevated in the first case and normal in the other; a fact that can be assessed, since the appearance of calcium in the urine has a multifactorial character. In fact, the greater intestinal absorption of calcium in some patients with PPH could justify this hypercalciuria, while the hypophosphatemia and hypercalcaemia itself would condition contradictory factors in absorption, mediated by $1,25(OH)_2 D_3$. If to this we add in some cases the decrease in renal glomerular filtration rate, due to hypercalcaemic nephropathy, the apparent paradox in the assessment of calciuria for the diagnosis of PPH could be justified. Magnesium: PTH acts on magnesium as it does on calcium, inducing an increase in renal tubular reabsorption and intestinal absorption, with greater mobilisation of magnesium in the bone compartment(48).

Decreases in magnesaemia were only seen in cases where there was another associated cause coro vomiting, acute or chronic magnesium repletion, which did not exceed 13% of cases.

The renal tubular components of magnesium are also not affected in PPH y only 16% of cases show a magnesium excretion rate higher than 0.100.

Acid-base balance: Among the functions of PTH is the reduction of proximal tubular reabsorption of bicarbonate, resulting in metabolic acidosis **(14).** In fact, this fact has been used for the differential diagnosis of hypercalcaemias, since PTH-dependent hypercalcaemias have a hyperchloremic acidosis, while hypercalcaemias of other origin have a normochloremic alkalosis (25).

However, in PPH this is complicated by the presence of other factors acting on the acid/base balance, such as renal insufficiency, increased bone resorption with mobilisation of other cations, citrates, sulphates, etc., so that overt hyperchloremic acidosis is found in only 30% of cases.

Biochemical markers of bone remodelling: Apart from the digestive and renal compartments, PTH acts preferentially on bone, leading to a stimulation of osteoclastic function with increased bone resorption. Only in some cases, especially in young subjects, has a certain osteoforming character been described, since PTH receptors are present in the osteoblasts **(37).**

In PPH we find alterations in bone remodelling, and, in fact, there are alterations in the formation markers in 53.8% of cases, coto total alkaline phosphatase (FAT), indicating that only half of PPH cases have active bone participation.

In order to be able to investigate the extent of the disease y possible visceral involvement, the determination of alkaline phosphatase isoenzymes (BAP) is useful. As we know, there are different tissue isoenzymes of BAP (bone, liver, post-hepatic, intestinal and placental origin). Therefore, the isoenzyme separation of FAT allows us to deduce whether there are multiple complications of tumours. For example, an increase in bone and liver fraction would indicate metastasis to the liver, and if posthepatic it would indicate any type of biliary obstruction.

The carboxy-terminal procollagen I peptide (PICP) and the amino-terminal propeptide of procollagen I (PINP) may serve as a useful index of bone formation, as we found a positive correlation with osteocalcin and a negative correlation with acid-tartrate resistant phosphatase.

Given that PTH preferentially induces bone resorption, it is logical to find greater alteration in the biochemical markers that measure bone resorption. Among these, fasting calciuria and the urinary hydroxyproline/creatinine ratio (Hp/cr), which was higher than 0.040 in 86.1% of patients, stand out in urine. The determination of plasma tartrate-resistant acid phosphatase (TRAP) and bone resorption index is also useful because of its affordability and cost-effectiveness **(14).**

Other more recent biochemical markers of bone resorption include pyriridoline (PYD), deoxypyridoline (DPD) as well as the umino-terminal (INTP) and carboxy-terminal (ICTP) telopeptides of type I collagen.)

Osteocalcin (BGP) is useful for measuring bone remodelling while providing evidence of bone formation. This marker is a useful index for the confirmation of PPH cases with bone participation.

The simultaneous determination of BGP y Hp/Cr ratio improves the differential diagnosis between the various forms of hypercalcaemia, since when both are elevated it points to the presence of PPH, while elevated Hp/Cr with low BGP suggests tumour hypercalcaemia. Hypercalcaemia with normal Hp/Cr o BGP indicates the absence of bone participation in PPH.

SPECIAL DETERMINATIONS

a) - PTH DETERMINATION

- Plasma: PTH is the definitive diagnostic method to distinguish PPH from other causes of hypercalcaemia. The specific biochemical diagnosis of PPH is made by determination of immunoreactive PTH, which is usually positive in up to 85% of surgically confirmed patients. The existing differences in plasma PTH activity, due to the heterogeneity of the antibodies used (which recognise carboxy-terminal fragments or half a molecule) explain the discrepancies between PTH values and parathyroid activity, explaining old published series, where up to 36% of surgically confirmed cases had normal PTH values. This data is nowadays more reliable with the immunoradiometric (IRMA) and immunochemiluminometric (ICMA) methods, which recognise the complete hormone (14).

b) OTHER AID

- - Fine needle aspiration: Fine needle aspiration biopsy has recently been incorporated for the diagnosis of parathyroid tumours whenever they can be localised with ultrasound, CT or MRI. Its reliability is 75% when the tumour is larger than 1 cm in diameter and preferably in adenomas, including mediastinal ones (26).

c) INSTRUMENTAL EXAMINATIONS

- - Radiology: Standard radiology for the study of bone participation in PPH includes chest X-ray (sometimes a mediastinal mass can be confirmed), lateral cranial X-ray (to visualise calcifications, calcifications, and possibly sella turcica pathology), simple abdominal and pelvic X-ray (to rule out renal-urological pathology and bone participation), hand X-ray and dental hard plate (to define subperiosteal resorption) (18).

- - Bone densidometry: Until not so long ago, the methods available for direct assessment of skeletal status were classical radiology y bone biopsy (50), but in recent years new techniques of a non-invasive nature have been developed for the measurement of bone mass "in vivo", either radiological (computed axial tomography, dual-energy X-ray absorptiometry [DXA]) or gammagraphic (single-photon absorptiometry, dual-photon absorptiometry). The accuracy of these methods varies from 4-6%, which is satisfactory compared to simple radiology where pathology is not detected until 30% of the bone mass has been lost (29).

Its use has become widespread with the assumption that decreased BMD is the main risk factor for fracture in osteoporosis, confirming its usefulness for the diagnosis and monitoring of bone damage in various metabolic diseases, as well as for the evaluation of the response to treatment (12).

HPP PREOPERATIVE LOCALISATION DIAGNOSIS.

Effective preoperative localisation helps to shorten surgical and anaesthesia time, so different imaging techniques have been used for the detection of abnormal parathyroid tissue (8,45). The efficacy of new localisation techniques, such as MIBI, is related to the anatomopathological finding, the anatomical localisation and the size of the tumour responsible.

Computed tomography (CT) is a problematic technique because of the iodinated contrast needed to distinguish between vessels and neck tumours; it has an average sensitivity of 63%(19). Magnetic resonance imaging (MRI), with a sensitivity of 74%, is costly and experience in parathyroid localisation is limited. High-resolution ultrasonography is an inexpensive and non-invasive method and is preferably used for preoperative localisation of abnormal parathyroid glands. It has a sensitivity of 34% to 92% and a false positive rate of 4% to 25%(23). These methods have preoperative sensitivity, so they are often used, after previous unsuccessful surgery, to localise abnormal parathyroid glands.

Nuclear medicine procedures are based on the use of isotopic markers directed at specific tissues. Of the various markers used, Tc-sestamibi(2-methoxy-isobutyl-isoni-trityl)(MIBI) is currently advocated, which allows localisation of abnormal parathyroid glands in patients with PPH. It is used alone o in combination with other radiopharmaceuticals (pertenectate o I) for subtraction studies. It is more sensitive for detecting adenomas than hyperplastic glands (58), with a sensitivity of 98-100% and a predictive value of 79% for solitary parathyroid adenomas, a sensitivity of 55-67% and a predictive value of 94% for hyperplastic glands, being more sensitive than high-resolution ultrasonography (57).

Chapter 3

<u>CONSERVATIVE TREATMENT</u>

A Consensus Conference has attempted to define asymptomatic PPH as well as its clinical management, study methods and treatment **(9).** b). - MEDICAL TREATMENT OF PPH

- General principles

In certain cases, medical treatment can be tried, increasingly consistent with the mild clinical manifestation of the disease, long survival and absence of secondary pathology in patients followed for years with this philosophy.

The indications for medical treatment, at least initially, are as follows: Calcaemia less than 11.5 mg/ml, absence of symptoms in direct relation to the disease o formal contraindication to surgical intervention.

The general principles of medical treatment of PPH are the same as for chronic hypercalcaemia of any etiology. It is important to suppress certain drugs, such as thiazide diuretics or lithium carbonate, which, while reducing urinary calcium excretion, have a direct effect on the parathyroid glands.

The **pharmacological treatment** of PPH includes the following rules:

- - <u>Substances that decrease PTH secretion.</u>

Several substances under study, including WR-2721, a drug used to protect normal tissues against the toxic effects of radiation and chemotherapy, have been shown to have a hypocalcaemic effect by inhibiting PTH secretion (16), and such antihormones may play a role in the medical treatment of PPH, tertiary hyperparathyroidism and in the management of recurrent parathyroid carcinomas (46).

- - <u>Substances that inhibit the effects of PTH.</u>

- Estrogens: The use of oestrogens y progesterone by inhibiting the resorptive effects of PTH have shown normalisation of calcaemia y bone mass gain in asymptomatic PPH, reduced treatment in postmenopausal women **(28).** Recently, oestrogen receptor modulators, including raloxifene, have also been used successfully to control the bone-lowering effect of hypercalcaemia in asymptomatic PTH cases **(59).**

- Bisphosphonates: Diphosphonates have been used both for the treatment of acute hypercalcaemia and for cases of inoperable carcinoma. We do not yet know the effect of second and third generation bisphosphonates on the chronic treatment of PPH **(21,43"47).**

- Phosphates: Administration of 1,0-2.5 grams of elemental phosphorus per day induces a decrease in calcaemia y calciuria which is often useful in cases of exclusive presentation of renal lithiasis. Oral sodium cellulose phosphate is effective in reducing calcaemia and calciuria **(40).**

Medical management of PPH should include calcaemia determination every six months y annual urinary calcium, creatinine clearance y bone densitometry (14) <u>Non-surgical parathyroid ablation.</u>

Parathyroid, cervical or mediastinal ablation, with contrast medium, hypertonic substances or alcohol, after angiographic tumour localisation with the introduction of flexible catheters facilitating selective injection, achieves long-term healing in 68% of cases. A number of transient complications have been reported (e.g. precordial pain, bradycardia, phrenic and vagus nerve dysfunction) and the only permanent complication is hypoparathyroidism in 6-11% of cases. Angio-ablation should not be performed if there is a strong probability of parathyroid carcinoma (21).

The success of this treatment depends on good preoperative localisation and should be reserved for patients at surgical risk, who have previously undergone surgery or who refuse open surgery(32).

SURGICAL TREATMENT

The treatment of PPH is exclusively surgical, especially in its symptomatic phases: hypercalcaemia or its visceral complications. As a general rule, a good surgeon is the best guarantee of a PPH solution (42).

a) .- INDICATIONS

Absolute indications for the surgical treatment of PPH are the existence of symptoms related to the disease (24). In 1990 the NIH established a series of surgical indications for asymptomatic PPH (TABLE V) **(9).**

In elderly patients with moderately elevated calcaemia, normal renal function and normal bone densitometry, periodic monitoring is usually more useful, reserving surgical exploration for symptoms or obvious signs (7).

b) TECHNIQUES AND RESULTS:

The surgical intervention requires careful haemostasis, general endotracheal anaesthesia and visualisation of the four glands, with intraoperative biopsies in case of doubt.

If an adenoma is detected preoperatively, a wide neck incision is usually not necessary, but a localised lateral incision. This saves surgical time by starting the dissection on the indicated side and quickly locating the large tumour. However, it is necessary to identify the other gland on that side coto normal, which avoids detailed dissection of the other side of the neck.

In cases of hyperplasia, all four glands should be localised with total excision of three of them and half of the remaining one, leaving 30-50 mg in the neck. In cases of carcinoma, confirmed intraoperatively, complete removal should be ensured, extended to possible metastases, avoiding local spread.

When the glands are not found on the first attempt, a supernumerary gland o in an ectopic situation, como in the thyroid o within a thymic remnant, should be suspected (42). In extreme cases, a median sternotomy should complete the surgical exploration. Another failure of surgery is the false diagnosis of PPH in familial hypocalciuric hypercalcaemia, which is a mandatory differential diagnosis.

<u>Operative mortality is</u> usually less than 1%.

d)   RECIDIVES

Recurrences of PPH are usually seen in 4-10% of operated adenomas. In cases of hyperplasia, the percentage rises to 13%, while in MEN, recurrences are usually as high as 30-44%.

The concept of "surgically cured" PPH has been altered by following these patients over time with periodic PTH measurements. The possible local spread of cells during surgical intervention (especially if the capsule is ruptured) may explain the spread of local foci of functioning tissue which is usually associated with local fibrosis adhering to neighbouring tissues. In other cases, up to 10% of patients who underwent surgery had elevated PTH levels for no known reason. This data makes it necessary to be cautious about the definition of curability of this disease **(41).**

RECOMMENDED BIBLIOGRAPHY

1. Albright F, CE Reifenstein. The parathyroid glands and metabolic bone diseaes: Selected studies. Williams & Wilkins. Baltimore. 1948 pp 125

2. Alvarez-Arroyo MV, Traba ML, Rapado A et al. Role of citric acid in primary hyperparathyroidism with renal lithiasis. Urol Res. 1992, 20: 86

3. Arnold A. Genetics basis of endocrine disease. 5. Molecular genetics of parathyroid gland neoplasia. J Clin Endocrinol Metab 1993, 77: 1108.

4. Bilezikian JP. Surgery or no surgery for primary hyperparathyroidism. Arch Int Med. 1985, 102: 402.

5. Bilezikian JP, R Marcus, MA Levine,ed. The parathyroids: Basic and clinical concepts. Raven Press. New York 1994,. pp 512

6. Broadus AE. Primary hyperparathyroidism viewed as a bihormonal disease process. Mineral Elect Metab. 1982; 8; 199.

7. Brothers TE, Thompson NW. Surgical treatment of primary hyperparathyroidism in elderly patients. Acta Chir Scand 1987; 175

8. Caixas A, M Puig. New techniques in the preoperative localization of hyperparathyroidism. Endocrinologia 1995, 42: 309

9. Consensus Development Conference Panel. Diagnosis and management of asymptomatic primary hyperparathyroidism: Consensus Development Conference statement. Ann Int Med, 1991, 114: 593.

10. Delellis RA. Tumors of the parathyroid glands. Atlas of Tumor Pathology. Third Series. Fascicle 6. Armed Forces Institute of Pathology. Washington, D.C., 1993, pp 176

11. Diaz Curiel M, Castrillo JM, Rapado A. Chloride/phosphorus ratio and hyperparathyroidism. Ann Int Med. 1977 87: 253

12. Diaz Curiel M, C. Turbi Disla, B. Perato, A. Rapado. Types of bone involvement in primary hyperparathyroidism. Rev Esp Enf Metab Oseas 1995; 4: 50

13. Diez Labajo A, Traba ML, Rapado A et al. Nephrolithiasis y participation osea in primary hyperparathyroidism. Relative role of vitamin D. Rev Clin Esp 1992,190: 238.

14. Endres DB, Villanueva R, Sharp CF, SingerFR. Immunochemilumi-nometric and immunoradiometric determinations of intact and total immunoreactive parathyroid. Performance in the differential diagnosis of hypercalcemia and hyperparathyroidism.Clin Chem 1991, 37:162.

15. Garton M, J Martin, A Stewart et al. Changes in bone mass and metabolism after surgery for primary hyperparathyroidism. Clin Endocrinol, 1995, 42: 493.

16. Glover D, L Riley, K Carmichael et al. Hypocalcemia and inhibition of parathyroid hormone secretion after administration of WR-2721 (a radioprotective abd chemoprotective agent). New Eng J Med 1983, 309: 1137.

17. Hamdy NAT, McCloskey EV, Brown CB, Kanis JA: Effects of clodronate in severe hyperparathyroidism bone disease in chronic renal failure Nephron 1990, 56: 6-12.

18. Hayes CW, WF Conway. Hyperparathyroidism. Radiol Clin North Am 1991, 29: 85.

19. Heath D.A. Localization of parathyroid tumours. Clin Endocrinol 1995, 43: 523.

20. Heath H, SF Hodgson, MA Kennedy. Primary hyperparathyroidism. Incidence, morbidity and potential economic impact in a community. New Eng J Med. 1980, 302:189.

21. Heller HJ, Miller GL, Erdman WA et al. Angiographic ablation of mediastinal parathyroid adenomas: local experience and review of the literature. Am J Med 1994, 97: 529

22. Kleerekoper M. A cure in search of a disease: Parathyroidectomy for nontraditional features of primary hyperparathyroidism. Am J Med, 1994, 96: 99

23. Krubsack AJ, Wilson S, Lawson T et al. Prospective comparison of radionuclide, computed tomographic, nosographic and magnetic resonance localization of parathyroid tumors. Surgery 1989, 106: 639

24. Lafferty FW, Hubay CA: Primary hyperparathyroidism: A review of the long-term surgical and nonsurgical morbidities as a basis for a rational approach to treatment. Arch Int Med. 1989, 149: 789.

25. Ljunghall S, J Rastad, G Akerstrom. Primary hyperparathyroidism: prevalence, pathophysiology, pertinent findings and prognosis. Bone and Mineral Research/8. JNM Hoersch, JA Kanis,ed. Elsevier. Amsterdam 1994,pp 1

26. MacFarlane MP, DL Fraker, TH Shawker et al. Use of preoperative fine-needle aspiration in patients undergoing reoperation for primary hyperparathyroidism. Surgery 1994, 116: 959

27. Mallette LE. Management of hyperparathyroidism in the multiple endocrine neoplasia syndromes and other familial endocrinopathies. Endocrinol Metabol Clin North America 1994, 23: 19.

28. Marcus R. Estrogens and progestins in the management of primary hyperparathyroidism.Endocrinol Metab Clin N Am 1987;18:715

29. Marcus R. Bone of contention: The problem of mild hyperparathyroidism. J Clin Endocrinol Metab 1995, 80: 720

30. Marx SJ, Familial hypocalciuric hypercalcemia. In Primer on Metabolic Bone Diseases and Disorders of Mineral Metabolism. 3ª edition. MR Marcus, ed. Lippincott-Raven. Philadelphia. 1996, pp 190

31. McBiles M, Lambert AT, Cote MG, Kim SY. Sestamibi parathyroid imaging. Seminars in Nuclear Med 1995, 25: 221.

32. McIntyre RC, DA Kumpe, RD Liechty. Reexploration and angiographic ablation for hyperparathyroidism. Arch Surg 1994, 129: 499

3 3 .Melton JL. Epidemiology of primary hyperparathyroidism. J.Bone Min Res, 1991, 6(Suppl 2): S25

34. Mundy GR, DH Cove, R Fisken. Primary hyperparathyroidism: Changes in the pattern of clinical presentation. Lancet 1980, 1:1317

35. Obara T, Fujimoto Y, Hirayama A et al.Flow cytometric DNA analysis of parathyroid tumors with special reference to its diagnostic and prognostic value in parathyroid carcinoma. Cancer, 1990, 65:1789

36. Perez Barba C. Solera J, Rapado A. Acute hyperparathyroidism. Rev Clin Esp. 1983, 171: 41

37. Piedra C, I Rios, J Ramos et al. The laboratory in the diagnosis of primary hyperparathyroidism. Rev Esp Enf Metab Oseas 1995, 4:44

38. Potts JT. Hyperparathyroidism and other hypercalcemic disorders. Advan Inter Med 1996, 41: 165

39. Rapado A. Arterial hypertension and primary hyperparathyroidism. Am J Nephrol 1986, 6(suppll): 49.

40. Rapado A, Castrillo JM, Esbrit P: Results of the administration of sodium cellulose phosphate coro medical treatment of primary hyperparathyroidism Med Clin 1984, 82: 702

41. Rapado A, MJ Molina, A Vazquez et al. Evolution of plasma parathyroid hormone values after surgery for primary hyperparathyroidism (Analysis of 86 cases followed for more than one year) Rev Esp Esp Enf Metab Oseas 1995, 4: 58

42. Rapado A, JM San Roman. Three hundred and nine operated cases of primary hyperparathyroidism: a shared experience. Rev Esp Enf Metab Oseas 1995, 4: 39

43. Reasner CA, Stone MD, Hosking DJ, Ballah A, Mundy GR: Acute changes in calcium homeostasis during treatment of primary hyperparathyroidism with risedronate J Clin Endocrinol Metab 1993, 77: 1067-71,

44. Resnick LM, Lewanczuk RZ, Laragh JH, et al. Parathyroid hypertensive factor-like activity in human essential hypertension. Relationship to plasma renin activity and dietary salt sensitivity. J Hypertension 1993, 11: 1235.

45. Rodriguez JM, Tezelman S, Siperstein AE, et al. Localization procedures in patients with persistent or recurrent hyperparathyroidism. Arch Surg 1994, 129: 870

46. Rosenblatt M. Peptide hormone antagonists that are effective in vivo. Lessons from parathyroid hormone. New Eng J Med 1986, 315: 1004.

47. Rossini M, Gatti D, Isaia G, Sartori L, Braga V, Adami S: Effects of oral alendronatr in elderly patients with osteoporosis and mild primary hyperparathyroidism J Bone Miner Res 2001, 16: 113-120,

48. Rude RK. Magnesium metabolism and deficiency. Endocrinol Metabol Clin North Amer. 1993, 22: 377.

49. Segre GV, Brown EM. Secretion, metabolism and circulating heterogeneity of parathyroid hormone. In: Primer on the metabolic bone diseases and disorders of mineral metabolism. 3ª edition. MJ. Favus, ed. Lippincott-Raven. Philadelphia, 1996,. pp 63

50. Serrano S, ML Marinoso. Bone histopathology in primary hyperparathyroidism, in: Patologia metabolica osea. S Serrano, J Aubia, ML Marinoso, ed. Sandoz. 1990, Barcelona, pp 155

5 1.Silverberg SJ, Shane E, Jacobs TP et al. Nephrolithiasis and bone involvement in primary hyperparathyroidism. Am J Med 1990;89:327

52. Solomon B, Schaaf M, Smallridge MD. Psycologic symptoms before and after parathyroid surgery. Am J Med 1994, 96: 99

53. Stefenelli T, Mayr H, Bergler-Klein J, et al. Primary hyperparathyroidism: Incidence of cardiac abnormalities and partial reversibility after successful

parathyroidectomy. Am J Med 1993, 95: 197

54. Thomas CG. The glands of Owen- A perspective on the history of hyperparathyroidism. Surgery 1990, 108: 939

55. Trigonis C,Hamberger B,Farnebo L et al.Primaiy hyperparathyroidism: Changing trends over fifty years. Acta Chir Scand 1983, 149: 675.

56. Vazquez A, MJ Molina. Molecular pathogenesis of hyperparathyroidism. Rev Esp En Enf Metab Oseas 1995, 4: 41

57.   Wei JP, GJ Burke, AR Mansbrger. Preoperative imaging of abnormal parathyroid glands in patients with hyperparathyroid disease using combi-nation Tc-99m-pertechnetate and Tc-99m-Sestamibi radionucleide scans. Ann Surg 1994, 219: 568.

58. Winzelberg GG. Parathyroid imaging. Ann Int Med 1987, 107: 64

59.   Zanchetta JR, Bogado CE: Raloxifene reverses bone loss in postmenopausal women with mild asymptomatic primary hyperparathyroidism J Bone Miner Res 16: 189-91, 2001

<u>**TABLE III**</u>

<u>**FAMILIAL ENDOCRINOPATHIES INCLUDING HPP**</u>

DOMINANT GENES	RECESSIVE INHERITANCE SYNDROMES
	Familial parathyroid adenomas
	Parathyroid adenomatosis with nephropaties y neuropathies
Multiple endocrine neoplasia 1	Parathyroid hyperplasia with parathyroid glands
Multiple endocrine neoplasia 2ª	
Parathyroid hyperplasia with intrathyroids	
fibro-osseous tumours of the jaw	Parathyroid hyperplasia with carcinoma o polyps of the colon
Isolated familial parathyroid adenomas	Parathyroid hyperparathyroidism with parathyroid carcinoma Isolated familial parathyroid hyperplasia.
Parathyroid carcinomas.	
Familial hypocalciuric hypercalcaemia with PPH	

<u>**TABLEIII**</u>

<u>**CHANGES IN THE CLINICAL PRESENTATION OF HYPERPARATHYROIDISM (%)**</u>

(452 CASES)

<u>1956-1965 1966-1975 1976-1985 1986-1990</u>

	1956-1965	1966-1975	1976-1985	1986-1990
№ OF CASES	**7**	**74**	**219**	**152**
OSTEITIS FIBROSA	72	14	5	2
LITHIASICS	14	46	42	30
HYPERCALCEMIC	14	22.9	19.3	16.7
H.P.P. AGUDO	0	0.1	2.7	1.3
ASYNTHOMATIC	-	8	21	40
NORMOCALCEMIC -		8	6	3
ENDOCRINE NEOPLASIA MULTIPLE		1	4	7

TABLEIII

BONE MINERAL CONTENT IN HPP ACCORDING TO DIFFERENT STUDIES

uthor№	A patients	Ano	Cortical	Trabecular	Technique
Silverberg et al	62	1990			SPA (radius) y DPA (CL, CF)
Martin et al	71	1990		NR	SPA (radio)
Wishart et al	28	1990			SPA (radius) y QCT (CL)
Abugasa et al	7	1990			SPA (radius) y DPA (CL)
Warner et al	28	1991		NR	SPA (radio)
Pfeilschifter et al	38	1992			SPA (radius) y DPA (CL, CF)
Minisola et al	62	1993	NR		DPA (radius y DXA (CL, CF)
Napal et al	30	1993	-		DPA (CL, CF)
Rico et al	29	1994			DXA (total body)
Diaz Curiel et al	107	1995			DXA (CL, CF, Radio)

CL: lumbar spine; **CF:** neck of femur; **NR:** not done; =: no change **Predominant bone^: CL:** trabecular bone; **Radius y CF:** cortical bone **SPA:** single photon absorptiometry; **DPA:** dual photon absorptiometry; **DXA:** dual X-ray absorptiometry;

BIOCHEMICAL VALUES IN 300 CASES OF HPP

Normal values Pathological findings of PPH

Analytical determinations

Range

Calcemia	mg/dl	9,1-10,5	>10,5
Creatinine accl	ml/min	80-125	<80
Nephrogenic cAMP % cAMP %			
nephrogenic cAMP		<63	>63
Serum PTH	pg/ml	10-80	>80
Calciuria	mg/24h	<250	>250
Ind.Exc.Calcium	mg/100 ml FG <0.175		>0,175
Serum phosphorus	mg/dl	2,7-4,4	<2,7
Serum Cl/P		25,4-40,0	>40
TmP/FG mg/100 ml FG		2,3-4,0	<2,3
Serum magnesium mg/dl		1.8-2.1	<1.7
Urinary Citrate/Cr *>0	.200		<0,200
Alkaline Phosphatase U.K.A.		2,3-10,3	>10,3
Osteocalcin	ng/ml	2,2-5,0	>6,0
Hyp/Cr	*	<0,030	>0,030
FATR	Ul/1	3,8-9,9	>9,9
Telopeptides	Pg/1	1,3-3,3	>3,2

* Both values expressed in mg/dl.
cAMP: cyclic adenosine monophosphate; TmP/GFR: renal phosphorus lintel;
K.A.U.: King-Amstromg units; GFR: glomerular filtration rate; FATR: tartrate resistant acid
 phosphatase; GFR: glomerular filtration rate

<u>**TABLAV**</u>

<u>**SURGICAL INDICATIONS FOR ASYMPTOMATIC PRIMARY HYPERPARATHYROIDISM**</u>

National Institute of Health Consensus Conference 1990

- **SERUM CALCIUM > 12 MG/DL**

- **URINARY CALCIUM EXCRETION > 400 MGRS/DAY**

- **BONE MINERAL DENSITY IN CORTICAL BONE < 2 Z-SCORE**

- **REDUCED CRESATININE CLEARANCE IN THE ABSENCE OF OTHER CAUSE**

- **AGE UNDER 50**

<u>**OTHER POTENTIAL SURGICAL INDICATIONS:**</u>

- **RECENT HISTORY OF FRACTURE IN THE ABSENCE OF MAJOR TRAUMA**

- **TRABECULAR OSTEOPENIA (Z-SCORE <2)**

- **VITAMIN D DEFICIENCY (25-OH VIT D <15NG/ML)**

- **PERIMENOPAUSAL WOMEN**

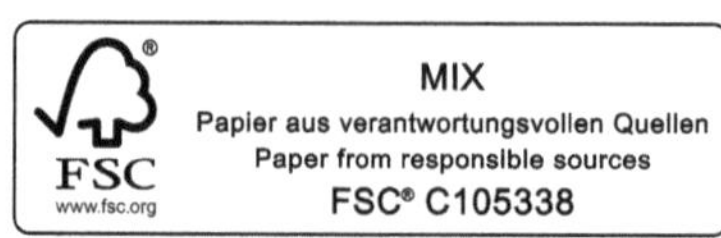

Printed by Books on Demand GmbH, Norderstedt / Germany